LET'S LOOK AT BODY SYSTEMS!

SASHA'S STRONG SKELETAL SYSTEM

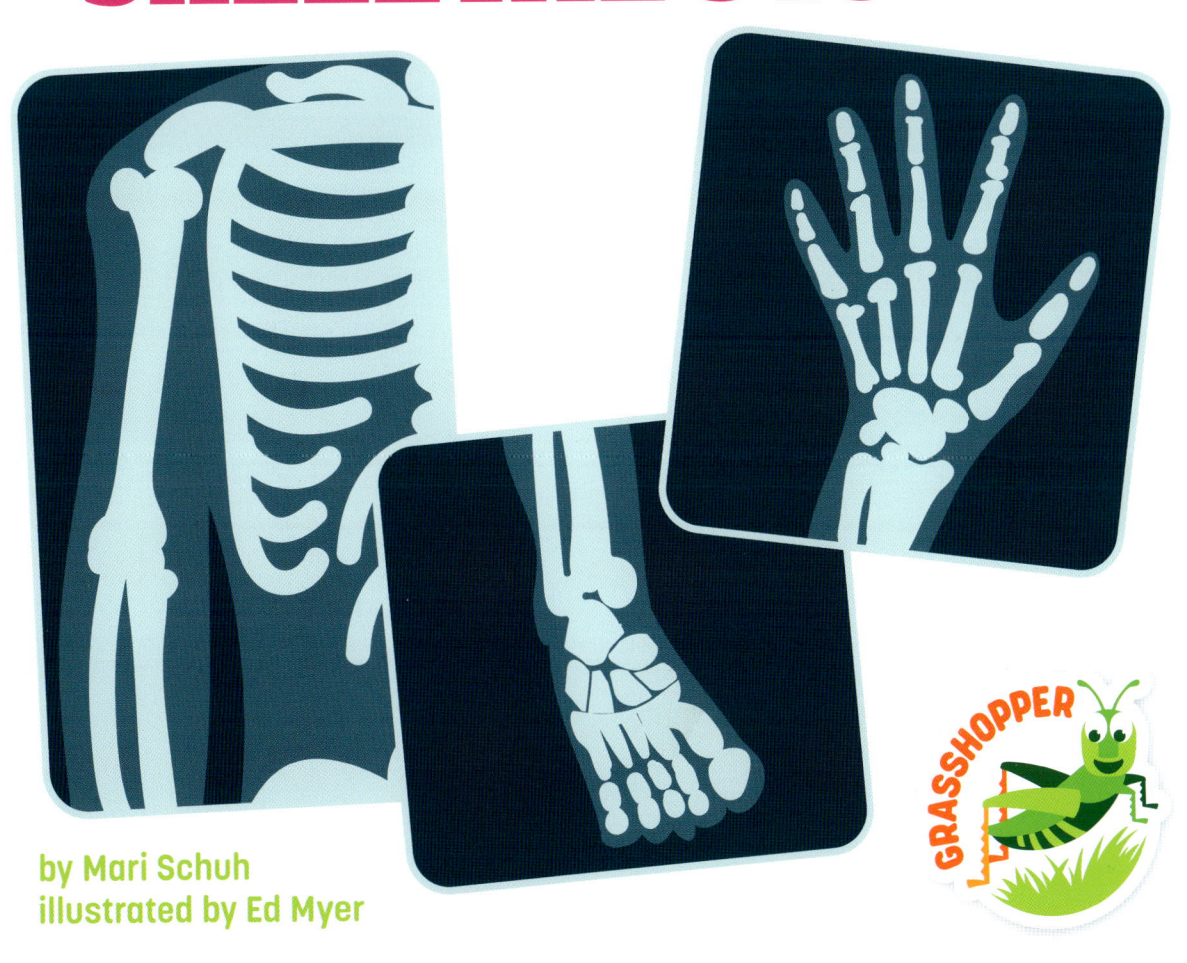

by Mari Schuh
illustrated by Ed Myer

GRASSHOPPER

Tools for Parents & Teachers

Grasshopper Books enhance imagination and introduce the earliest readers to fiction with fun storylines and illustrations. The easy-to-read text supports early reading experiences with repetitive sentence patterns and sight words.

Before Reading
- Discuss the cover illustration. What do they see?
- Look at the glossary together. Discuss the words.

Read the Book
- Read the book to the child, or have him or her read independently.
- "Walk" through the book and look at the illustrations. Who is the main character? What is happening in the story?

After Reading
- Prompt the child to think more. Ask: Think about how you move your body each day. What does your skeletal system help you do?

Grasshopper Books are published by Jump!
5357 Penn Avenue South
Minneapolis, MN 55419
www.jumplibrary.com

Copyright © 2022 Jump! International copyright reserved in all countries. No part of this book may be reproduced in any form without written permission from the publisher.

Library of Congress Cataloging-in-Publication Data

Names: Schuh, Mari, author. | Myer, Ed, illustrator.
Title: Sasha's strong skeletal system / by Mari Schuh; illustrated by Ed Myer.
Description: Minneapolis, MN: Jump!, Inc., [2022]
Series: Let's look at body systems! | Includes index.
Audience: Ages 7-10
Identifiers: LCCN 2021038019 (print)
LCCN 2021038020 (ebook)
ISBN 9781636906539 (hardcover)
ISBN 9781636906546 (paperback)
ISBN 9781636906553 (ebook)
Subjects: LCSH: Human skeleton–Juvenile literature.
Human physiology–Juvenile literature.
Classification: LCC QM101 .S349 2022 (print)
LCC QM101 (ebook) | DDC 611/.71–dc23
LC record available at https://lccn.loc.gov/2021038019
LC ebook record available at https://lccn.loc.gov/2021038020

Editor: Jenna Gleisner
Direction and Layout: Anna Peterson
Illustrator: Ed Myer

Printed in the United States of America at Corporate Graphics in North Mankato, Minnesota.

Table of Contents

On the Move	4
Where in the Body?	22
Let's Review!	23
To Learn More	23
Glossary	24
Index	24

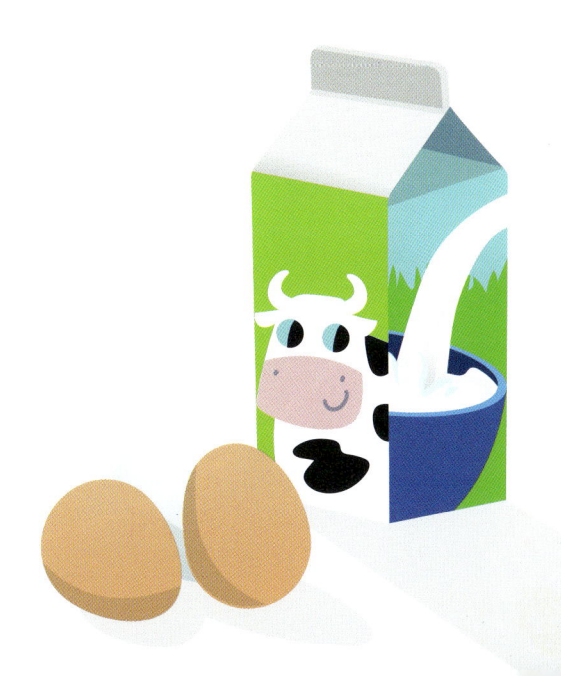

On the Move

"Hey, Dad! Watch this!" Sasha says.

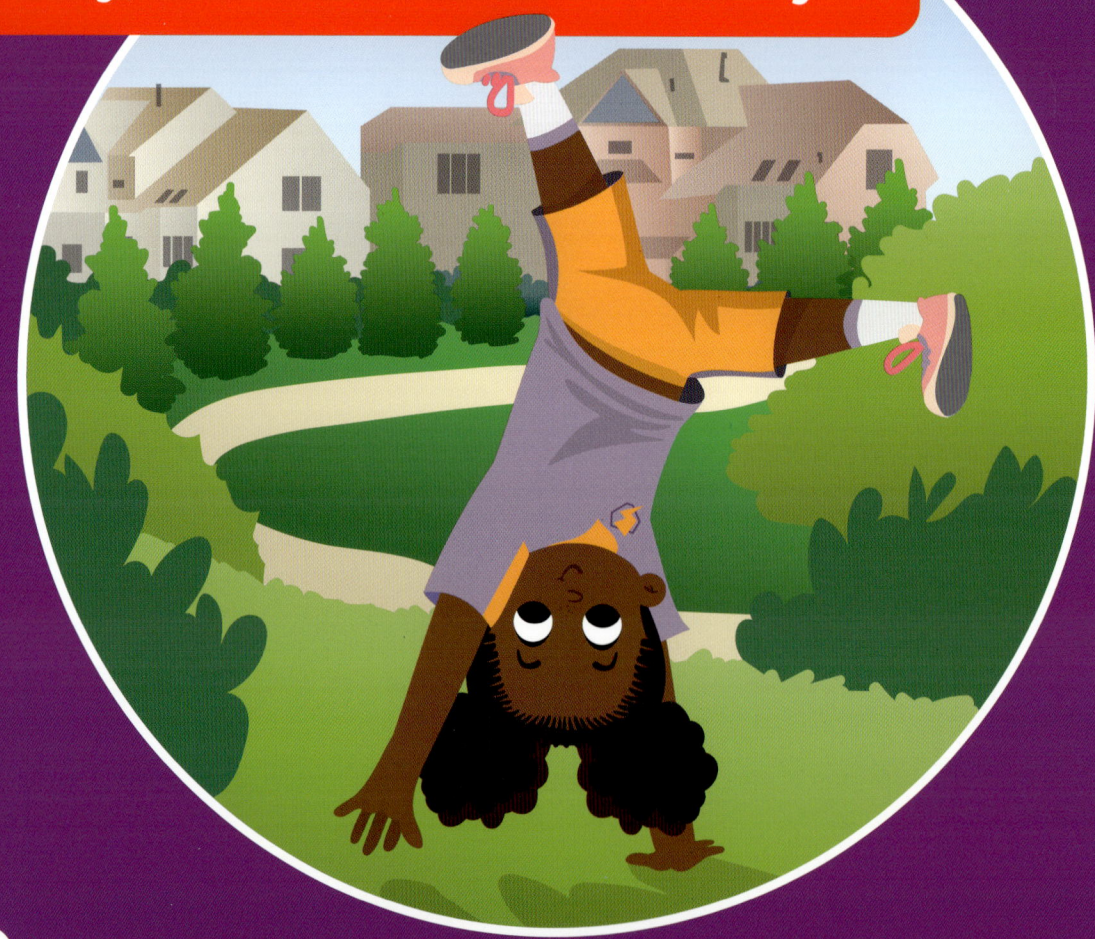

"How does my body help me move?" Sasha asks.

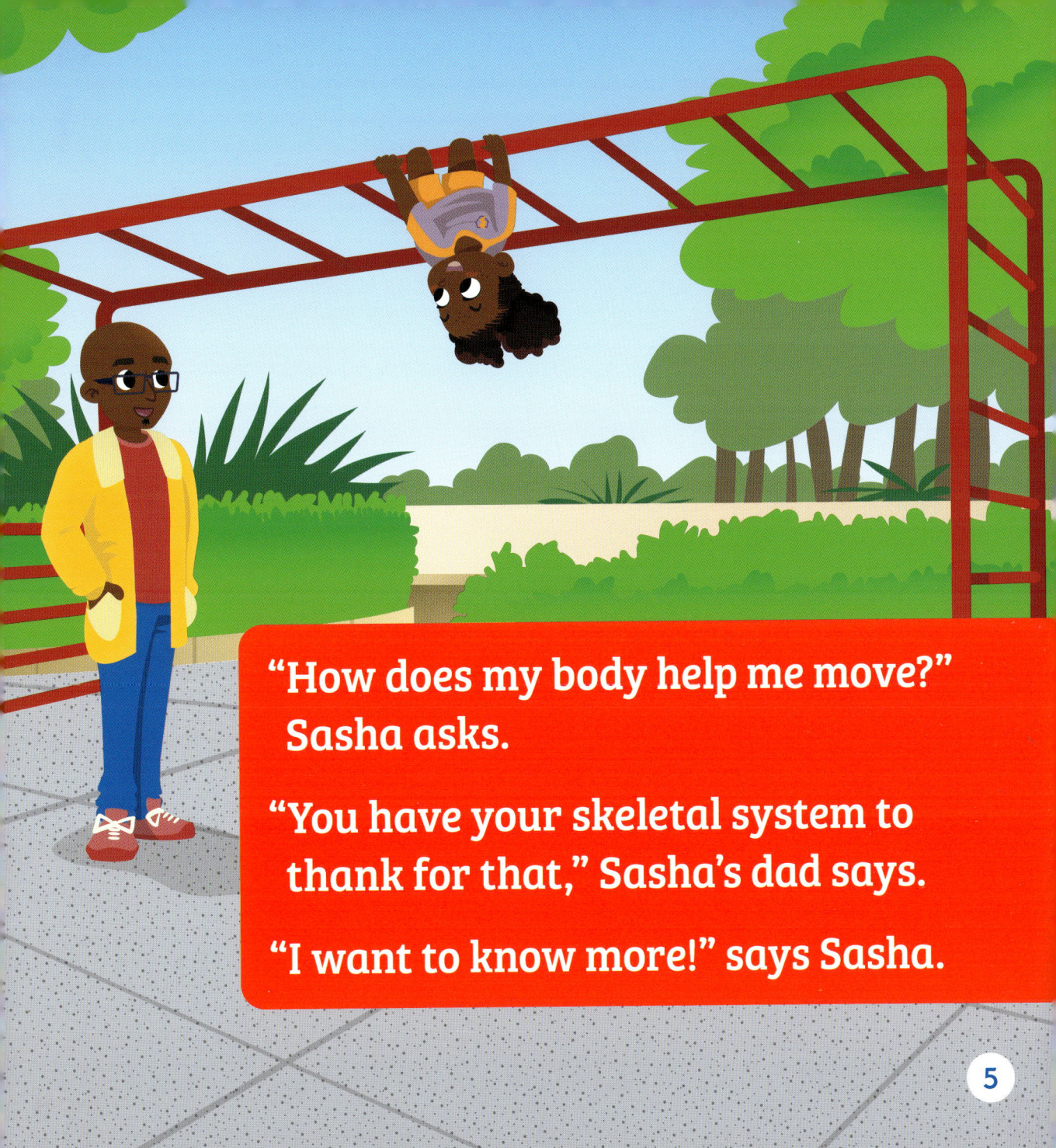

"You have your skeletal system to thank for that," Sasha's dad says.

"I want to know more!" says Sasha.

"From your head to your toes, your body has 206 bones! You can feel them. See?" says Sasha's dad.

"Bones are hard and strong. Together, they make up your skeletal system. Your skeleton gives your body shape. Without it, your body would be like jelly!" he says.

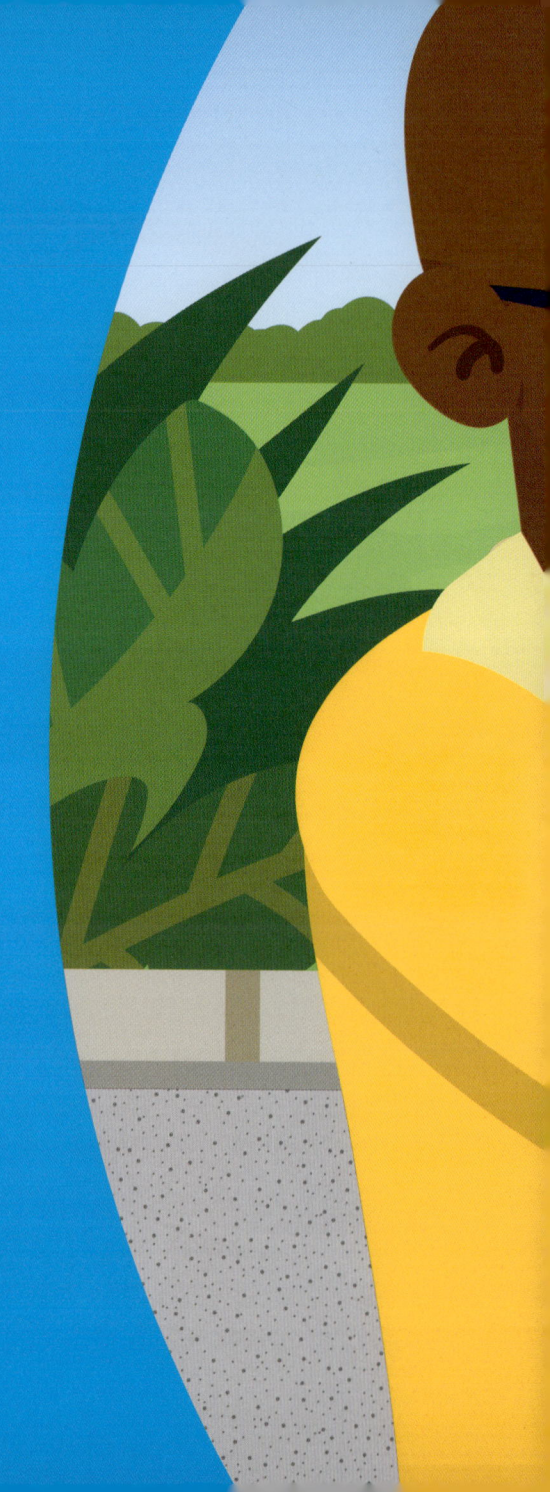

7

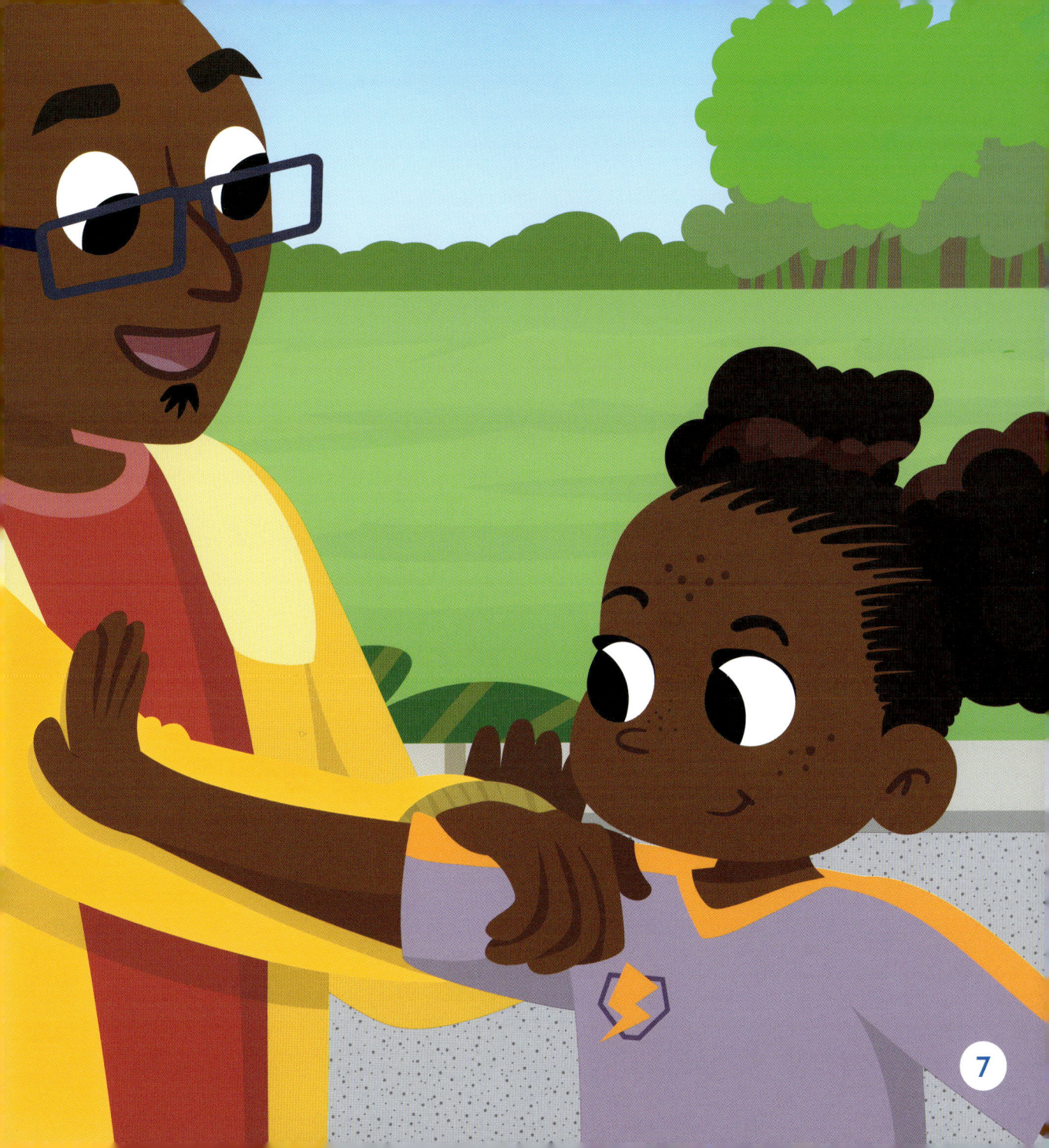

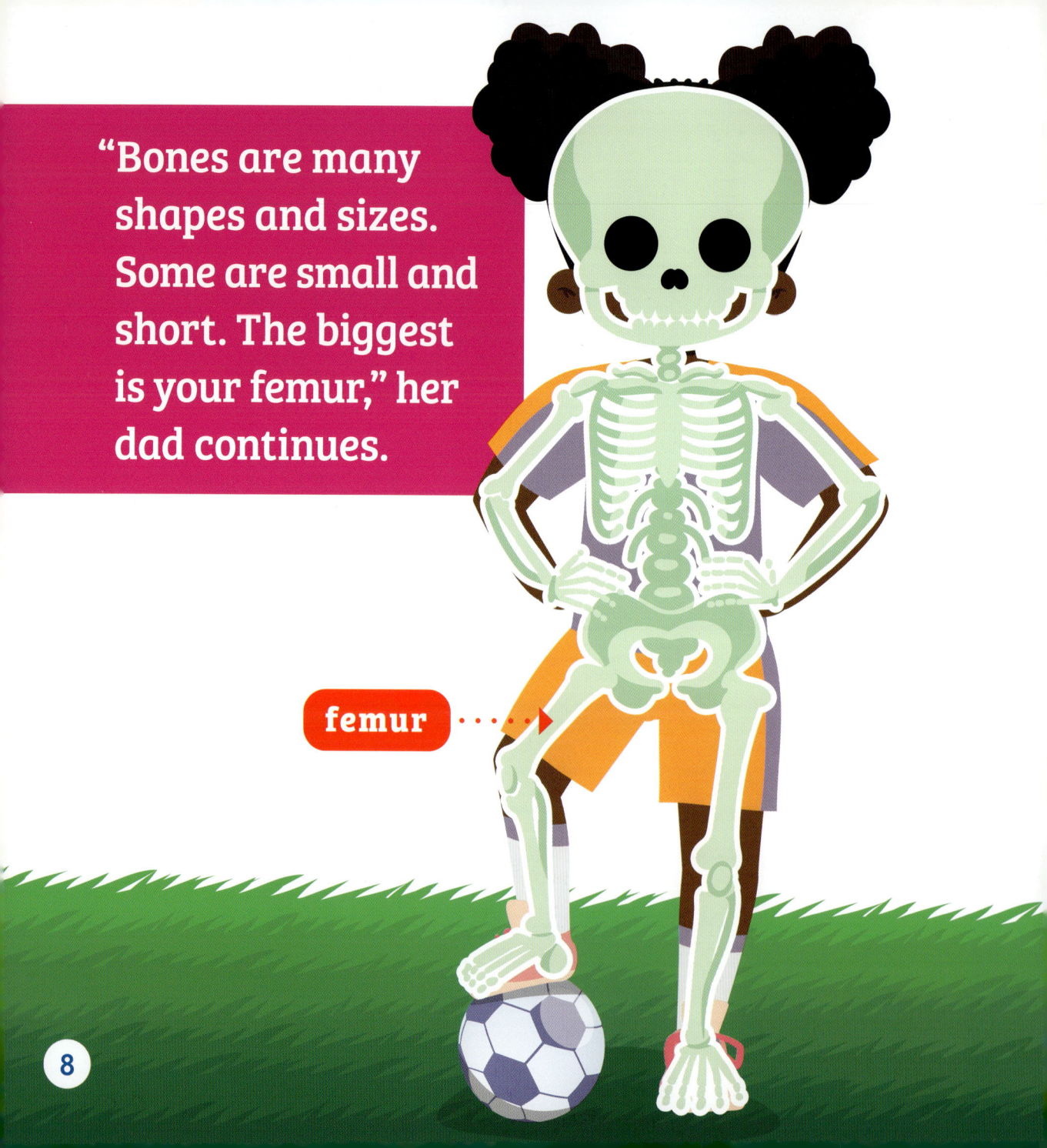

"Bones are many shapes and sizes. Some are small and short. The biggest is your femur," her dad continues.

femur

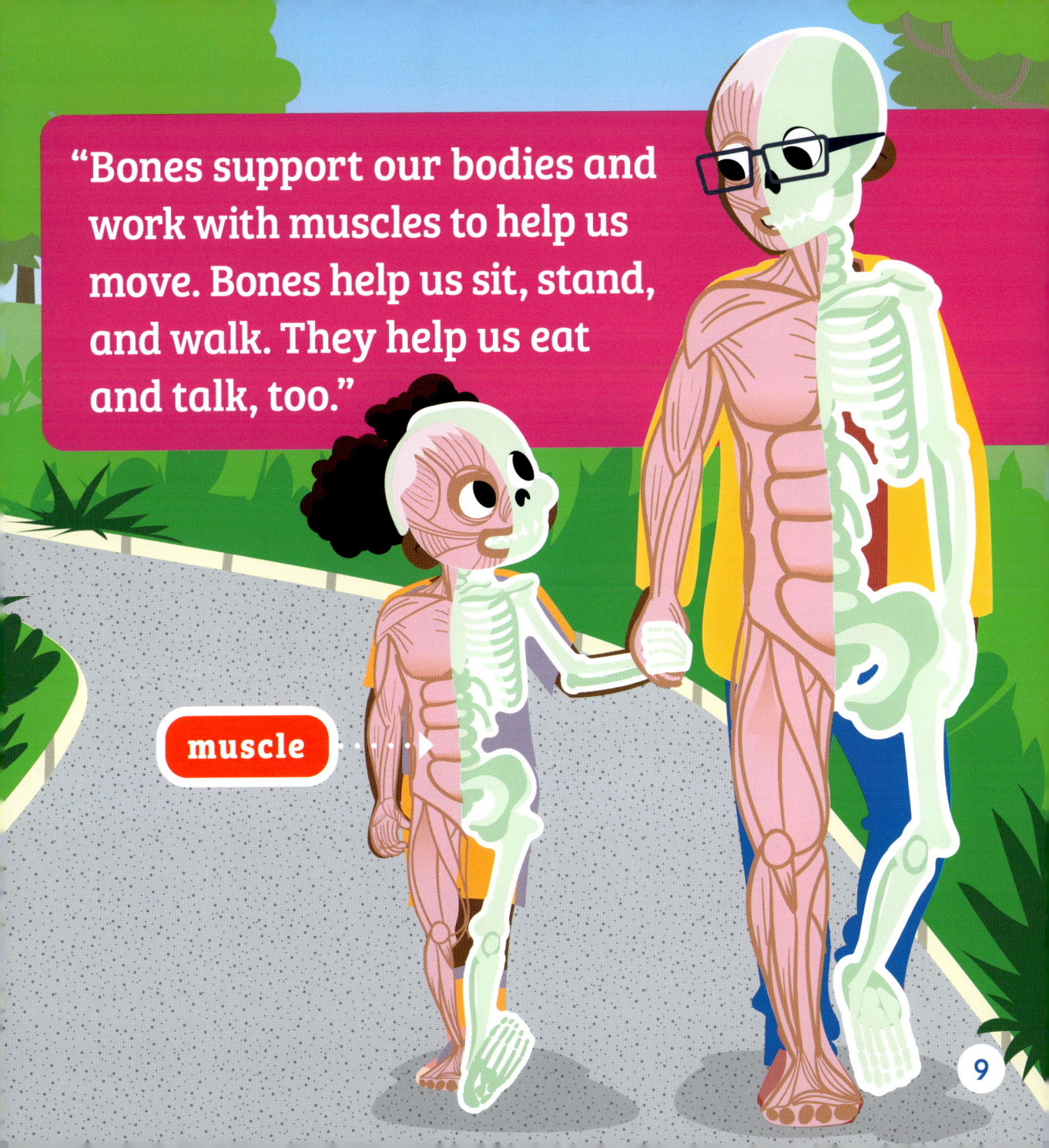

"Bones support our bodies and work with muscles to help us move. Bones help us sit, stand, and walk. They help us eat and talk, too."

muscle

"What about when I play soccer?" Sasha asks.

"Your bones help you run and kick the ball. They also keep your organs safe. Your ribs form a cage to protect your heart and lungs. Your skull protects your brain," he says.

skull

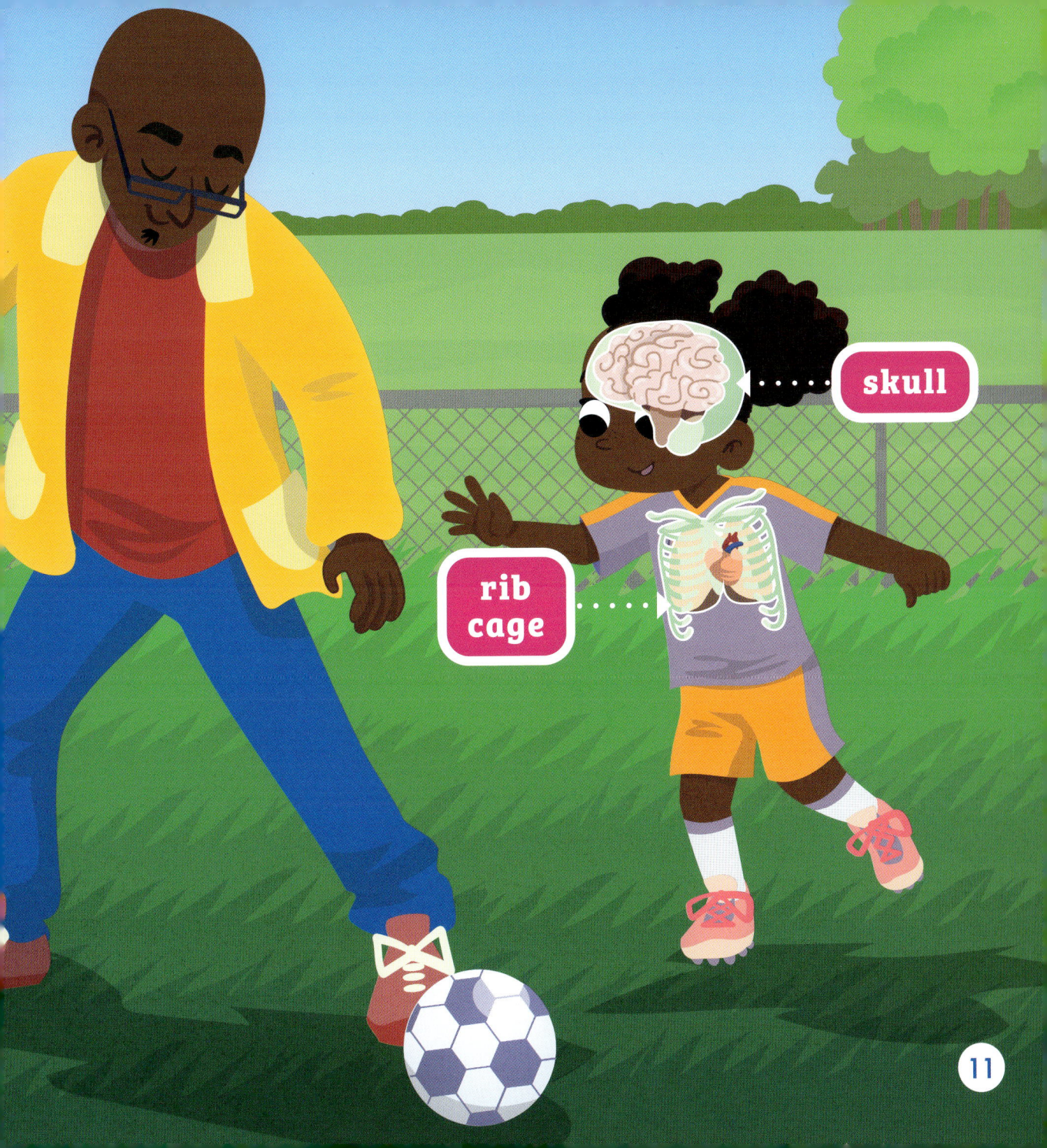

rib cage

11

"But how do my bones help me move? And how are they connected?" Sasha asks.

"Many parts work together," Sasha's dad says. "Bones meet at joints. Joints are made of fluid and cartilage. Tough bands of tissue called ligaments connect bones. Tendons connect muscles to bones. These are stretchy to help you move."

tendon

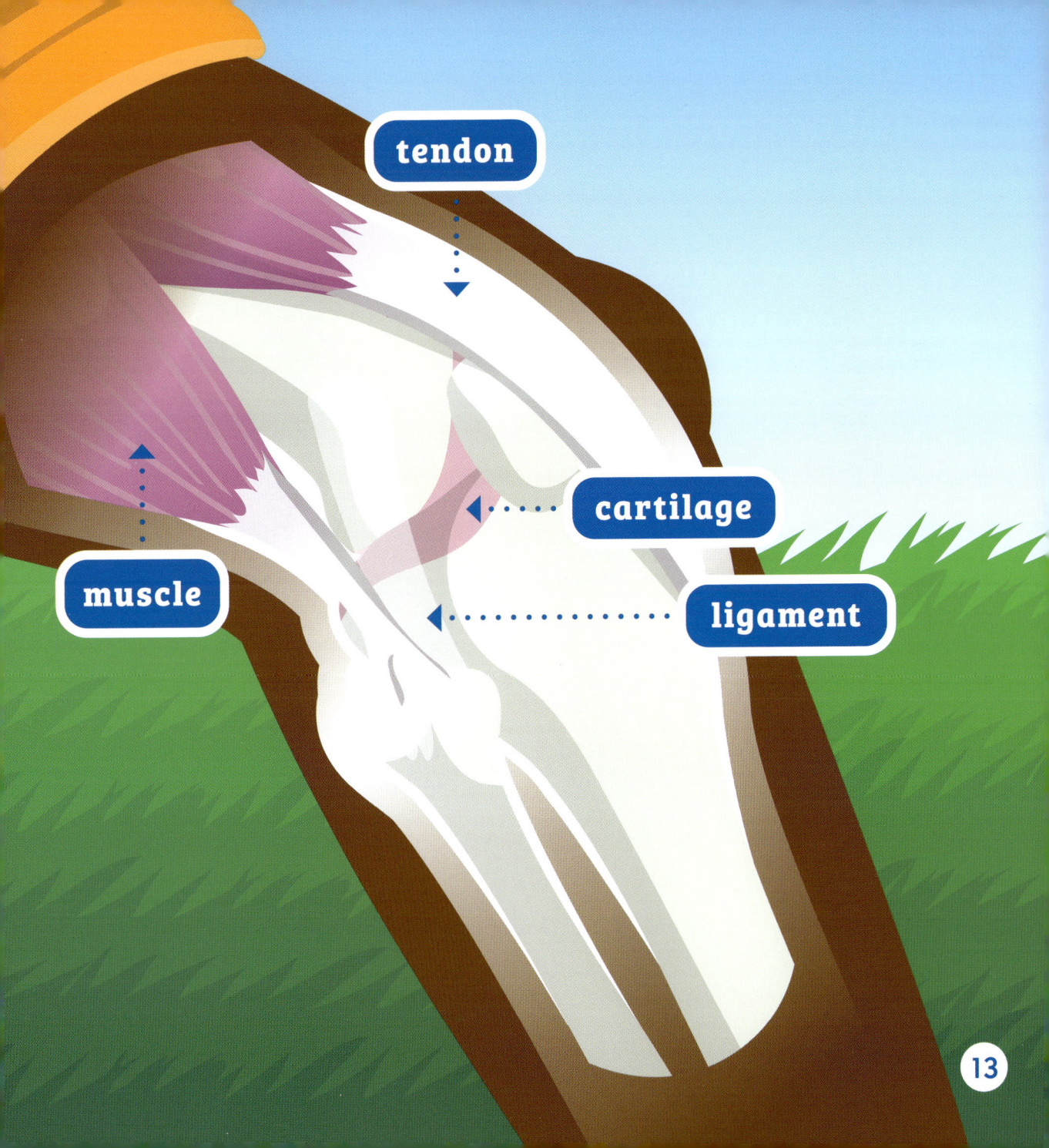

muscle

cartilage

ligament

13

"What are bones made of?" Sasha asks.

"Bones are made of calcium, protein, and water. Periosteum covers the outside. Under that is a hard layer called compact bone. Spongy bone is inside. It has spaces filled with bone marrow," her dad says.

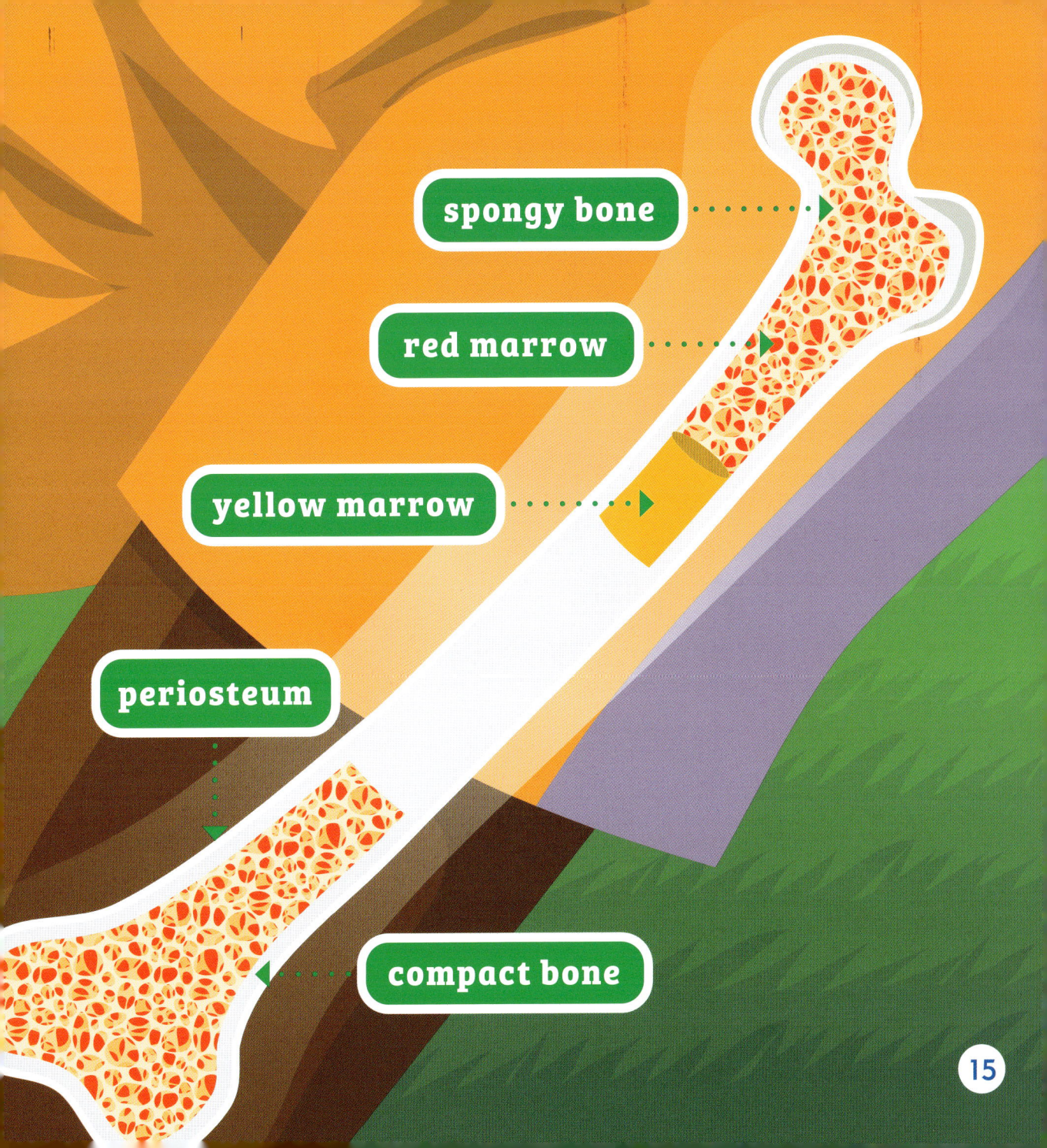

- spongy bone
- red marrow
- yellow marrow
- periosteum
- compact bone

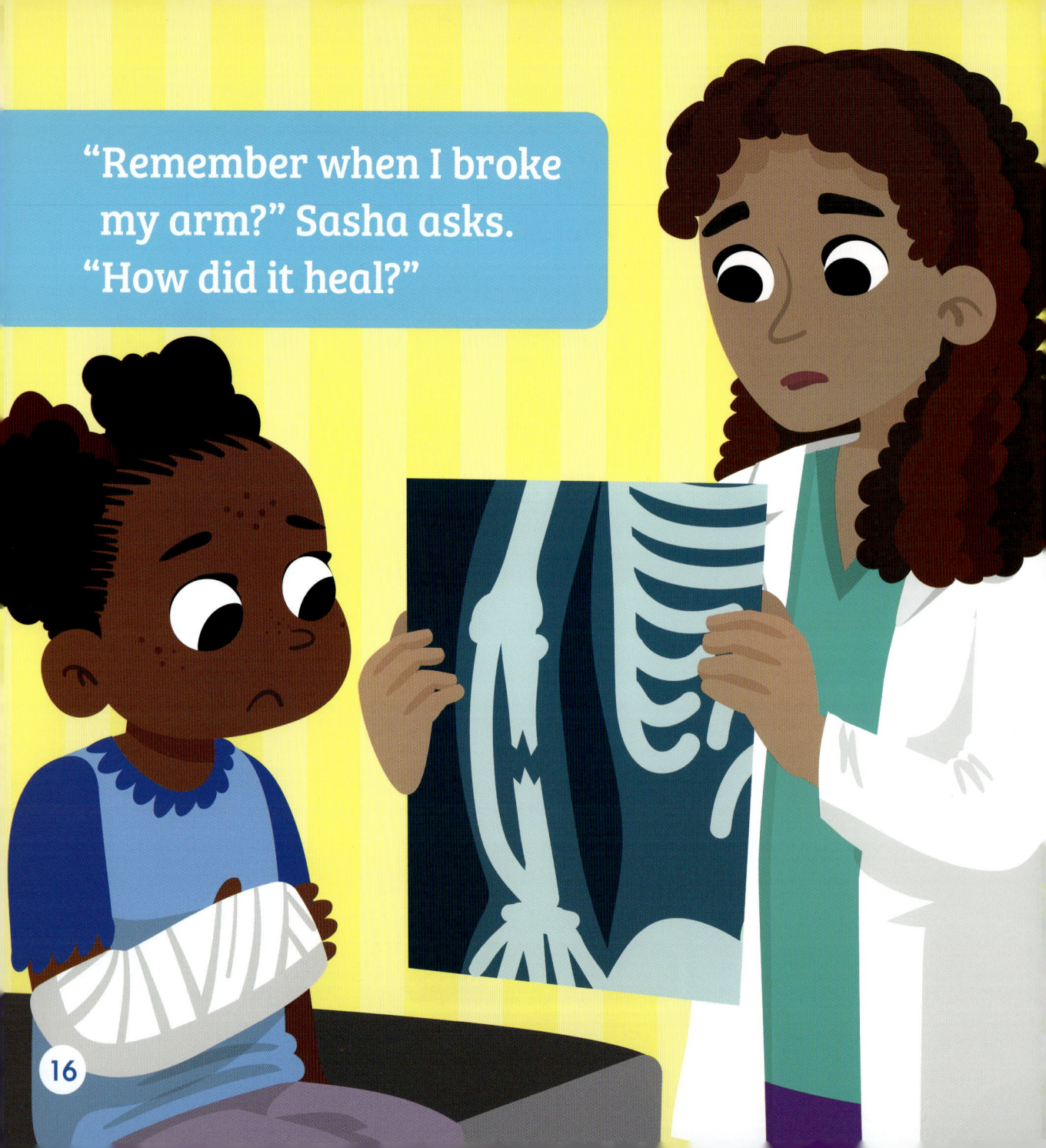

"Remember when I broke my arm?" Sasha asks. "How did it heal?"

bone

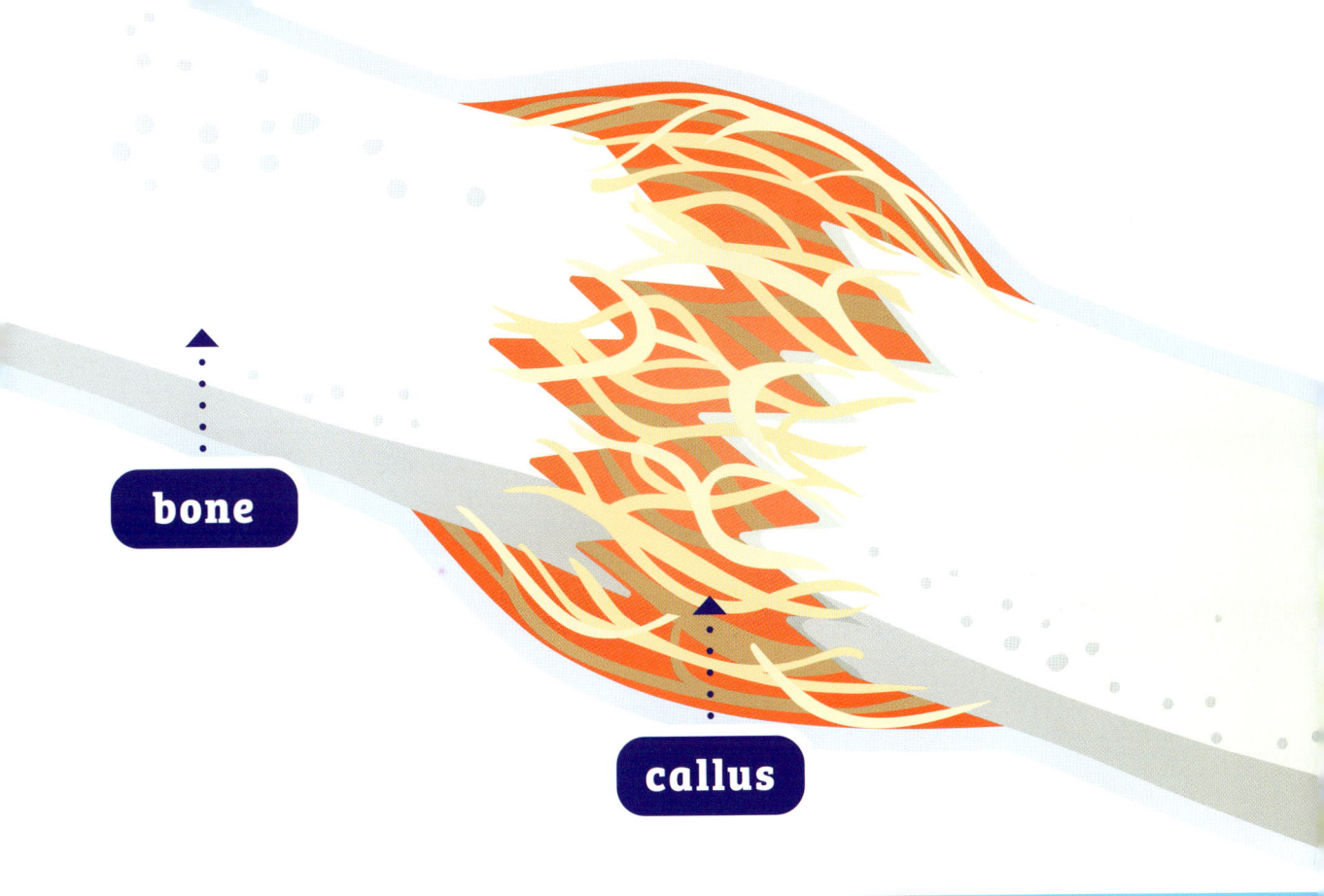

callus

"A soft callus formed around your bone. It helped join the broken pieces. The callus got harder, and new bone started to grow," her dad explains.

"I hope I never break another bone!" Sasha says.

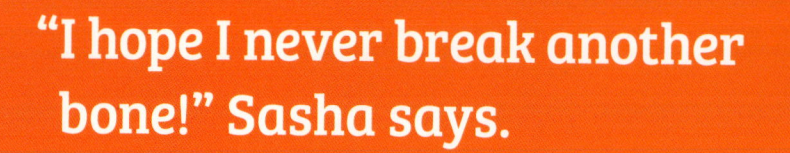

"That's why we eat healthy foods!" her dad says. "Foods with calcium and vitamin D help build strong bones. Staying active helps, too."

19

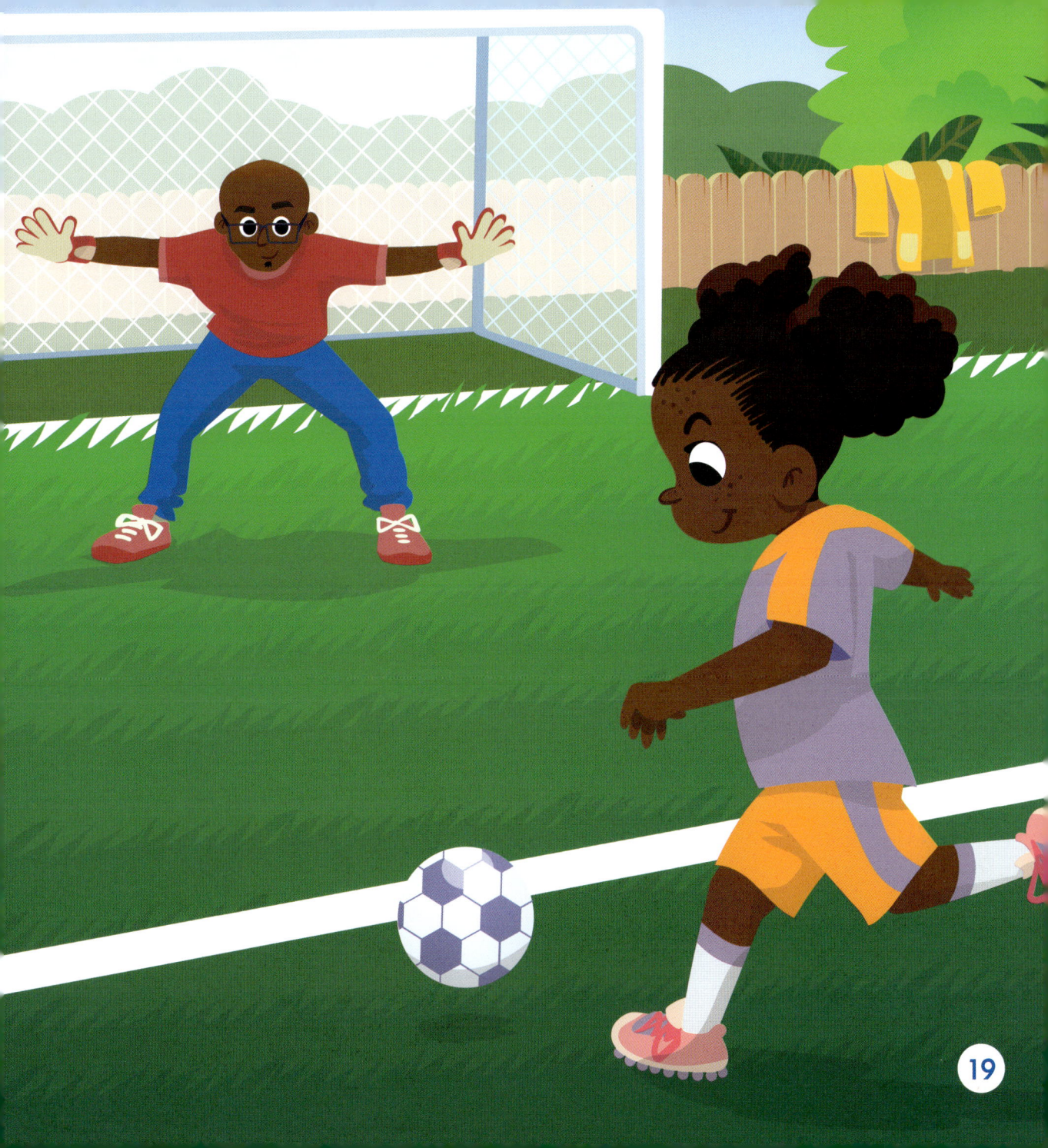

"We use our bones every day. So it's important to take care of them every day, too. That's why we wear safety equipment. It protects our bones!" Sasha's dad says.

"Our bones are healthy and strong!" says Sasha.

21

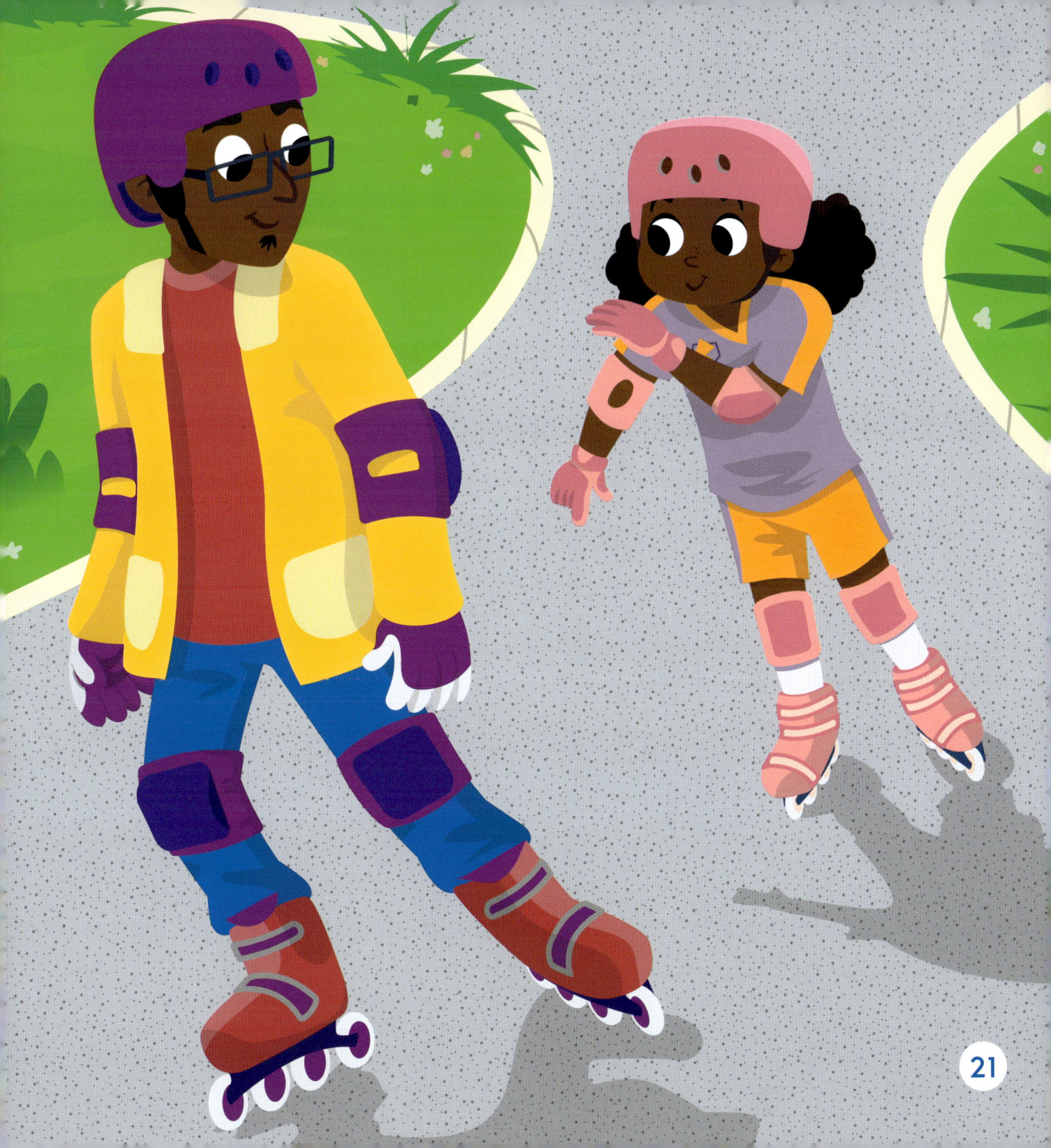

Where in the Body?

What are some of the main bones of the skeletal system? Take a look!

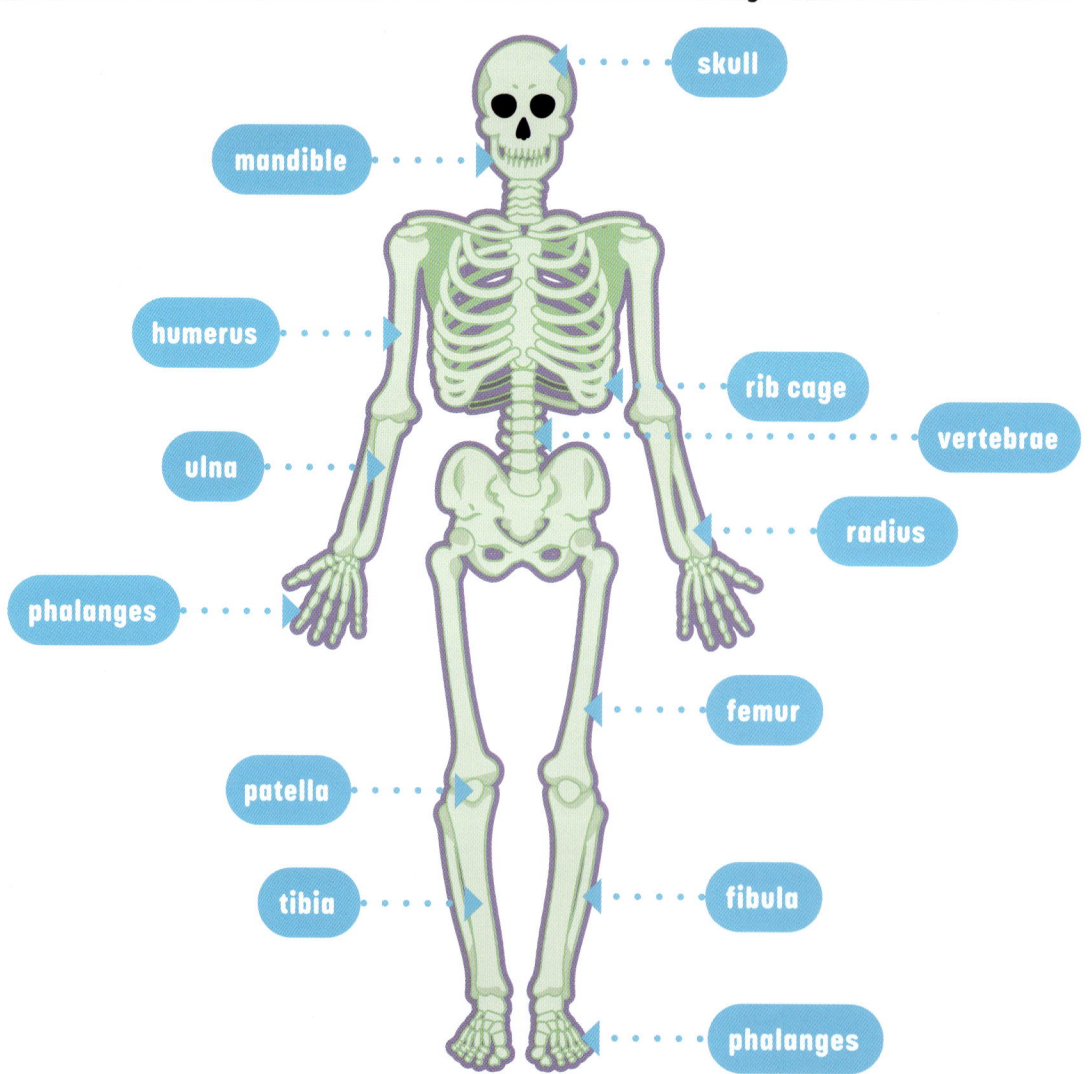

- skull
- mandible
- humerus
- rib cage
- vertebrae
- ulna
- radius
- phalanges
- femur
- patella
- fibula
- tibia
- phalanges

Let's Review!

Foods with calcium and vitamin D help build strong bones. You can eat these foods to keep your bones healthy and strong!

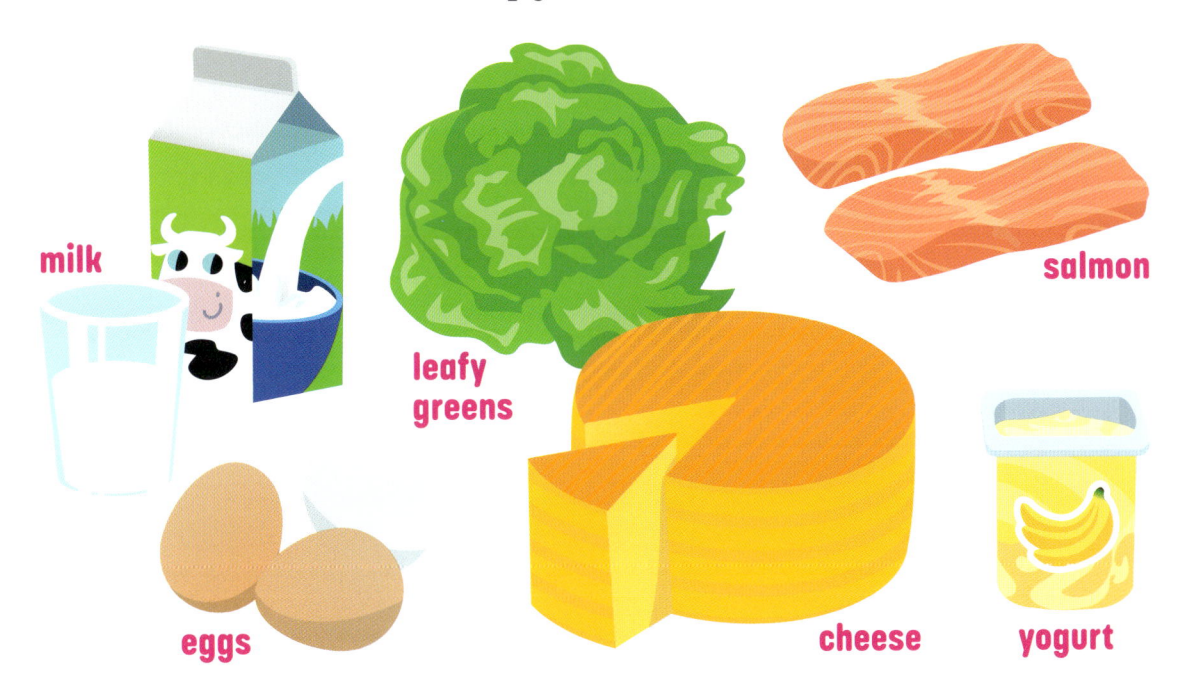

milk

leafy greens

salmon

eggs

cheese

yogurt

To Learn More

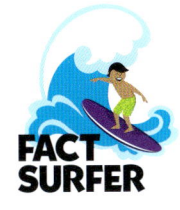

Finding more information is as easy as 1, 2, 3.

1. Go to www.factsurfer.com
2. Enter "**Sasha'sstrongskeletalsystem**" into the search box.
3. Choose your book to see a list of websites.

Glossary

calcium: A soft mineral found in bones and teeth.
cartilage: Strong, rubbery tissue that connects bones.
joints: Places where two or more bones meet.
ligaments: Tough bands of tissue that connect bones.
marrow: A soft substance inside bones in which blood cells are made or where fat is stored.
muscles: Tissues in the body that can contract, or shorten and tighten, to produce movement.
organs: Parts of the body that do certain jobs.
periosteum: A thin membrane that covers bones.
protein: A substance found in all living animal and plant cells.
skeleton: The bones that support and protect the body.
tendons: Stretchy, strong tissues that connect muscles to bones.

Index

bone marrow 14
broke 16, 17, 18
calcium 14, 18
cartilage 12
compact bone 14
femur 8
ligaments 12
muscles 9, 12

organs 10
periosteum 14
ribs 10
skeleton 6
skull 10
spongy bone 14
tendons 12
vitamin D 18